Nourish and Nurture

Overlooked Ingredients and Empowering Poetry
for Pregnancy, Breastfeeding, and Motherhood

*For the best of
health! Erin
love,*

Erin L. O'Reilly

Healthy Nourishment, LLC
Saint Louis, Missouri

Nourish and Nurture: Overlooked Ingredients and Empowering Poetry for
Pregnancy, Breastfeeding, and Motherhood
© 2023 Erin L. O'Reilly

First printing: 2023

This book was created with the help of an Editwright team.
Visit editwright.com for more Editwright works.

Developmental editing by Andrew Doty
Copy editing by Karen L. Tucker
Book design by Peggy Nehmen, n-kcreative.com
Photography by Brea Youngblood

Published by Healthy Nourishment, LLC
Saint Louis, Missouri

Erin L. O'Reilly shares her experiences and knowledge as a public speaker for
classes, workshops, seminars, and special events. To contact the author about
speaking at an event, visit ErinLOReilly.com.

Library of Congress Control Number: 2023904414

ISBN:
Paperback: 978-1-7344388-2-6
E-book: 978-1-7344388-3-3

BISAC
HEA044000 HEALTH & FITNESS / Breastfeeding
MED036000 MEDICAL / Health Policy
HEA028000 HEALTH & FITNESS / Health Care Issues

To All Mothers

Contents

Introduction

I am a public health nurse and a lactation consultant who has been working with mothers and babies for over 30 years. My first interest was nutrition, and I had entertained going to school to become a dietitian but went to nursing school instead. Through an associate degree nursing program, I could get out of school sooner and start earning an income. During my early years of hospital nursing, after seeing the unpleasant, painful, and costly aspects of illness (tertiary care, or treating illnesses rather than preventing them), I changed course. I turned to maternal/child, community health, and primary preventive health care nursing, where I could promote healthy lifestyle behaviors and work to prevent illnesses from occurring. I obtained a bachelor of science in nursing (BSN), then a master of science in nursing research (MSNR) in community health nursing and started my work with mothers and babies in prenatal care, labor and delivery, postpartum care, and home visits with young families. I taught childbirth education and breastfeeding classes for over 20 years.

As a mother, I had challenges with breastfeeding my own son and got involved with La Leche League to get the support I needed for breastfeeding. I became a La Leche League Leader in 1999 and was certified as an International Board Certified Lactation Consultant (IBCLC) in 2000. I came back around to nutrition through my work in lactation and worked with dietitians in the Women, Infants, and Children (WIC) program for 13 years, helping babies get the best nutrition through breastfeeding. My interest in maternal nutrition grew as I saw how important nutrition is to support the health and stamina needed for pregnancy, motherhood, and breastfeeding. Good maternal nutrition also reduces the too-common complications of pregnancy, birth, and breastfeeding.

In this book, I cover some important "nutrients" (I am using this term in a broad sense) that are overlooked and often lacking in the heavily processed American diets and unnatural lifestyle. The nutrients I focus on are vitamin D, zinc, magnesium, and fiber. These nutrients are all important for maternal health and well-being. The fifth "nutrient" is oxytocin, an important hormone that affects pregnancy, birth, breastfeeding, and infancy.

These nutrients are the "nourish" part of the book. They are all good for the maternal oxytocin system, which is crucial for maternal and infant health. The best way to get these nutrients is through healthy nutrition, sun exposure, and skin-to-skin/hands-on care rather than vitamin pills, but sometimes supplements are needed. Most pregnant women do take prenatal vitamins, but current prenatal vitamins are not ideal for these specific nutrients.

I am including some recipes at the end of each chapter. The foods I have chosen for these recipes are good not only for each specific nutrient covered in that chapter, but also for the other nutrients I discuss in the other chapters.

I love poetry also, so I have combined my interests in this book of *Nourish and Nurture*. My poems, the "nurture" part of this book, are meant to be enlightening in a pleasurable way about the importance, beauty, and empowerment of breastfeeding for both mother and baby. This book also includes some photos of breastfeeding mothers and their babies along with their words of inspiration.

I hope the information on nourishment and the nurturing poems and photos inspire pregnant and breastfeeding mothers to enjoy getting and giving (breastfeeding) the best nutrition for the best health. I also hope readers gain knowledge and empowerment and take pleasure in this book of nourishment and nurture.

NOTE: I am not a doctor or a dietitian, and I am not recommending any specific nutrient intake or amounts. I am, as a public health nurse/lactation consultant, trying to shed some light on nutrients that are often overlooked by our medical care system and are often deficient due to our American eating habits. I discuss these nutrients as they relate to pregnancy, breastfeeding, motherhood, and infancy. I do not suggest that anyone take large doses of vitamins; rather, the best way to get nutrients is from fresh foods that are grown and prepared in a natural way, without the use of herbicides, antibiotics, artificial chemicals, heavy processing, or overcooking. I want to educate pregnant women and mothers so they can make healthy, informed choices with regards to nutrition, perinatal care, and infant nutrition. If a mother or infant is suspected or found to have insufficient levels of nutrients, then she should discuss this with her own health care providers.

Nourish

Nutritional history in the United States

M uch of the processed food industry in the United States was built up to feed the soldiers in combat during World War II. At the end of the war, instead of being dismantled, this profitable industry was marketed to the general public instead. Highly processed foods lack many nutrients. Nutrients can be added back in to processed foods but are not easily bioavailable and often lead to imbalances with other nutrients. Our modern lifestyle also does not allow enough time for food growing, informed shopping, meal preparations, or mindful eating, all of which affect our digestion and nutrient assimilation.

Eating fresh foods as close to the way they grew in nature (in other words, unprocessed) has been one of the main concepts guiding the work of La Leche League. The La Leche League (LLL) founders started saying this back in the 1950s when LLL was founded, but also when the popular diet in the United States was to get the mother out of the kitchen by serving "fast foods" that were highly processed. During this time, TV dinners, fast-food chains, and drive-throughs became popular in the United States. These and other processed/chemicalized/overcooked foods stripped of their nutrients have caused the malnutrition that underlies most chronic diseases. These foods have the macronutrients of fats, proteins, carbohydrates, and calories but lack the equally important micronutrients. "You are what you eat," as the saying goes, and good nutrition is one of the most important aspects of good health! The LLL founders have been right about nutrition all along and deserve recognition for steering mothers back toward eating healthy and natural foods rather than highly processed fast foods.

Pregnancy, birth, breastfeeding, and motherhood

We women have the ability and responsibility (if we choose it) to bear, birth, and breastfeed a baby: our progeny, humankind's future. This is amazing! Our ability to adapt and change to grow and feed a baby is unique and endows us with talents, but it also burdens us with extra needs, work, and responsibilities that deserve research, support, and funding. Male-dominated modern life and obstetrics have stepped in to "help," but this help comes with a loss of control and often just ends up throwing additional barriers and pain, topped off with medical expenses, into our paths. Maternal nutrition is basically ignored, or, if it is given any public health attention and funding, such as through WIC, it is very regimented, dairy heavy, and uses very little fresh foods in its supplemental program. Even though WIC encourages breastfeeding, it also provides too much infant formula and not enough breastfeeding support.

The heavy focus on medically oriented obstetric care in the USA does not allow time, attention, or funding for the basic nutritional needs of the mother and child. Yet poor nutrition is involved in 80% of all illnesses and also in poor perinatal outcomes. Nutrition therapy is ordered only when a health problem is diagnosed, such as gestational (pregnancy-related) diabetes or too little or too much weight gain. By that time, it is too late, and the problem is already entrenched; the stage is set for future health problems that could have been avoided if good nutrition had been tended to before or, at least, early during pregnancy.

Pregnancy increases the need for healthy foods, calories, and nutrients. This makes pregnancy an opportune time to screen for nutritional adequacy and test for nutrient levels. Healthy levels of nutrients lower the risks of pregnancy-related illnesses and also ensure that the fetus receives needed nutrients.

Infancy, pregnancy, and breastfeeding are times in a person's life that have great influence on health in later life. They are times when the door is open to influence immunity, metabolism, and growth in a healthy or unhealthy manner. This opportunity door closes when infancy, pregnancy, and breastfeeding end. This is why good nutrition is *critical* during infancy, pregnancy, and breastfeeding! Every pregnant and breastfeeding mother deserves nutritional therapy and guidance specific to her—her needs, characteristics, cultural influences, skin color, environmental and geographical influences, family and social history, and dietary influences. Obstetrical care in the USA is not currently stepping up to do this.

Maternal malnutrition not only negatively affects the mother and fetus during pregnancy but also manifests through intergenerational effects via poor outcomes in children's growth; neurodevelopment; and cognition, cardio-metabolic, pulmonary, and immune functions. Metabolic disease (obesity, diabetes, high blood pressure, and fertility problems) is becoming very common, and poor nutrition during pregnancy, inappropriate weight gain during pregnancy, and not breastfeeding all increase the risk of metabolic disease seriously for both mother and child. I discuss this in my other book, *The Recipe for Breastfeeding Support in America.*

Primary preventive health care begins with good nutrition—nutrition for the mom before and during pregnancy and breastfeeding, and nutrition for the infant and child —and sets the stage for future health. By not giving pregnant women and mothers the primary preventive nutritional care they need, American medical care is missing an opportunity to decrease gestational diabetes, preeclampsia, premature births, fetal growth problems, breastfeeding problems, and other problems that afflict American mothers and babies for as long as they live.

This lack of *primary preventive nutritional* care (focused on health promotion and disease prevention) from the health/medical care system forces women to seek the information they need for themselves. I hope this book will help you with this task. We are what we eat, and what goes in dictates output—how our bodies and minds perform. Humans have survived and thrived on fresh foods from nature. It is only in the past 100 years that we have started eating heavily processed and chemicalized foods. During this same time, chronic disease has replaced acute infectious diseases as the dominant health care problem in the USA, especially metabolic diseases such as obesity, high blood pressure, fertility problems, and diabetes. Poor nutrition is heavily involved in all these diseases.

Each of the chapters in this book will discuss:

- The nutrient and its roles and importance in pregnancy and breastfeeding
- Symptoms, conditions, and problems related to deficiencies of the nutrient
- Current obstetrical (OB) policy and practices regarding nutrient assessment and supplementation
- Healthy nutrient levels through diet and/or lifestyle
- Foods and recipes that are high in the nutrient

For more information about nutrients, visit my website, erinloreilly.com. Poems, breastfeeding photos, and mothering/breastfeeding messages are included in the back of this book in the "Nurture" section.

I will begin with vitamin D in Chapter 1. Chapter 2 covers zinc, Chapter 3 covers magnesium, Chapter 4 is about fiber, and Chapter 5 describes massage as it relates to oxytocin, a very important hormone for pregnancy and breastfeeding. These important but often ignored nutrients deserve as much attention and assessment as folic acid, iron, and calcium are given during a pregnancy! Prenatal vitamins are a poor source for zinc, magnesium, vitamin D, and fiber because they are less bioavailable, absent, and/or combined with noncompatible nutrients, which can decrease their absorption. Prenatal vitamins also are not regulated and can have variable amounts of a nutrient or even not have certain nutrients included at all. Yet prenatal vitamins are treated like they are the answer to all nutritional problems—they aren't! The best nutrition comes from fresh food and a healthful diet. Vitamins are supplemental and need to be regulated for nutrient adequacy!

Dietary assessment by a registered dietitian (RD) and blood-level testing would be good to do for all pregnant and breastfeeding women, and even for women planning a pregnancy. You can ask your OB doctors for a referral to a dietitian, if one is not offered, and/or blood tests if you think you might have a deficiency. Most insurances will cover these assessments with a doctor's order. Pregnancy is often a time when mothers are inspired to improve their nutrition, so getting an appointment with an RD for a thorough assessment and education is a wonderful way to start on your journey to becoming a healthy mother! If you qualify for WIC, you will automatically be assigned to an RD and will have the nutritional assessment, along with supplemental foods, given to you. If you qualify for Medicaid, then you qualify for WIC. Kids can qualify for WIC also until six years of age.

Vitamin D

Vitamin D (called the "sunshine vitamin" but actually a steroid hormone) is important for so many biological functions: immune and cardiovascular health, digestive microbiota, muscles and nerves, bones, skin, mental health, fertility, maternal and fetal health, and protection against cancers. Associations exist between D insufficiency and many diseases, including tuberculosis, psoriasis, multiple sclerosis, inflammatory bowel disease, metabolic disease (including diabetes), high blood pressure, heart failure, myopathy, rickets, breast cancer, and other cancers. Respiratory illnesses, including COVID-19, are also more serious if there is a D deficiency. Vitamin D is definitely important for more than just skeletal strength. The levels of vitamin D needed to prevent many other diseases are higher than what has been historically recommended. As we modern humans have become less connected to the outdoors, we also tend to suffer from lack of sunshine and lower D levels. Vitamin D is now the subject of much research and revisions to the levels needed for healthy living.

Importance during pregnancy and breastfeeding

Specifically related to pregnancy, D affects fetal neural development and differentiation and contributes to the regulation of
around 900 genes, including the oxytocin receptor gene, which
I will discuss in Chapter 5. D is important for placental function,
maternal cardiovascular health, hormonal balance, blood sugar
regulation, fetal calcium homeostasis, and bone mineralization,
which all influence fetal and maternal well-being, and is crucial
for a healthy pregnancy and breastfeeding.

Not only is D an important nutrient, but it is also a prohor-
mone and helps to activate other hormones such as oxytocin,
serotonin, and vasopressin, which are important to pregnancy
and childbirth. Magnesium, which I will discuss in Chapter 3,
is also required for the receptor of oxytocin to function well and
is important to keep in balance with D.

Symptoms, conditions, and problems related to deficiencies

The following conditions are related to inadequate levels of D:
higher blood pressure in pregnancy and preeclampsia, preterm
birth, poor fetal growth and lower birth weights, decreased bone
mineralization of fetus, increased risk of maternal depression,
gestational diabetes, higher levels of inflammation during pregnancy, uterine muscle inefficiency during birth, higher C-section
rates, milk production problems, and low transfer of D to infant.
These are all very serious complications!

Babies who are born with low D levels due to the mother's
low prenatal levels also are at greater risk for many health problems related to deficiency of D: premature birth and stunted
fetal growth resulting in low birth weight, poor weight gain and

growth in infancy, delayed motor development, rickets, muscle weakness, aches and pains, fatigue, fractures, and depression.

Problems with D occur not only due to poor nutrition, but also our lack of healthy outdoor sunlight exposure because of the indoor lifestyle of modern living. Even the temperature of your skin can affect D levels, and our skin temperatures are going down with sedentary, indoor lifestyles! Many people now have normal temperatures in the 97-degree Fahrenheit range rather than 98.6, which is historically considered the average human temperature.

Humans are a *part of and dependent on nature*—as the song says, "we are stardust"—and we need nature for our survival and health. We need sunlight in healthy proportions, and we aren't getting enough, so D levels are low in many people. It is estimated that *at least* 40% of Americans have too low D levels, with much higher deficiency levels in darker-skinned people, those who do not have access to safe or healthy outdoor spaces, those who live in northern latitudes, low-income families who can't afford healthier but more expensive foods, vegans, heavily clothed people who don't get sun exposure, and older, diabetic, and overweight people.

Current prenatal policy and practice

The American College of Obstetricians and Gynecologists (ACOG) recommends testing only pregnant women who are at increased risk of D deficiency, yet with so many reasons that women can be deficient, as I stated above, it would be better if *all* pregnant and breastfeeding women were screened. Screening should also include an assessment by a registered dietitian (RD) for nutritional intake through diet and lifestyle (to assess for sun exposure) as well as through lab studies. Adding a D test to prenatal blood labs is easy and inexpensive compared to treating D deficiency–related problems. D screening during pregnancy is an important public and primary preventive health care measure!

Pregnant and breastfeeding women are NOT routinely screened for D levels, which puts the baby at risk for low D levels, since low levels during pregnancy and breastfeeding means the baby will also suffer with low levels. OB health care practitioners have differing opinions and practices regarding levels of testing, supplementation, and maternal circulating D. Prenatal vitamins only have 400–600 international units (IU) of D in them, but the more recent doses recommended for *routine* supplementation (versus supplementation for deficiencies or for pregnancy) are up to 2,000 IUs, so why is the D in prenatal vitamins so low? D levels in vitamins also need to be geared to the time of year and environment to accommodate for less sun exposure in winter months and more northerly locations.

Better quality research and updated policies are needed to inform OB health care providers and pregnant women on this issue. Pregnant women can ask for D screening if it is not offered. It is easy to add this blood screening level to your other prenatal labs, which should be covered by insurance with a doctor's order. You can also ask for a referral to an RD for nutritional/lifestyle assessment and lab screening of blood levels, and then to be treated with appropriate supplemental D if your levels are low.

Assessment, sources, and supplementation

• *DURING PREGNANCY*

With around 40% of people being deficient in D levels and pregnancy increasing the need for vitamin D, it can be assumed these factors present greater risks for prenatal deficiencies. If the current supplementation levels of D for nonpregnant adults is 1,500–2,000 IUs for the maintenance of adequate blood levels, then the increased needs of pregnancy mean the prenatal vitamin D levels of 400–600 IUs are too low and extra vitamin D will be needed during pregnancy, especially if deficiency is suspected. If deficiencies are found, then supplementation is a good idea, and this should be discussed with your health care provider.

If your health care provider does not screen you or refer you to a dietitian for assessment, and you think you might be deficient due to lifestyle, skin color, or dietary issues, you can get tested and purchase vitamin D supplements over the counter to take in addition to your prenatal vitamins, but it would be more thorough and accurate to be screened and treated in response to your specific levels. Vitamin D levels are expressed two ways—nanograms per milliliter (ng/mL) and nanomoles per liter (nmol/L)—which is confusing but needs to be recognized for adequate interpretation.

• *DURING BREASTFEEDING*

Current pediatric practice is to supplement all breastfed babies with vitamin D daily. It is disappointing that vitamin D supplementation for breastfed infants is routine policy but screening pregnant and breastfeeding mothers is not routine! This is an example of what I call a "mothering inequity," and it points to the fact that OB policies need to be updated on this issue since it implies that all breastfed babies start with too-low vitamin D levels from their mothers.

NOTE: Formula has D supplementation added, so the recommendation is for breastfed infants to be supplemented with extra D. This recommendation assumes that the mother's milk is low in D levels in addition to the assumption of low transfer of D during pregnancy due to inadequate prenatal levels of D.

This routine supplementation for babies is hard to do, as many babies don't take medicines well and caregivers are too busy just feeding and caring, so it often gets forgotten. A more personalized approach is to screen and treat before or at least during pregnancy to ensure the fetus got a good dose through pregnancy. Then, if low during breastfeeding, instead of the baby being supplemented, the mother can take 6,400 IUs per day to increase the levels in her milk, which will help increase her levels also. This can easily be monitored—blood tests are a cheap public health measure compared to treating expensive illnesses associated with vitamin D insufficiency.

Healthy levels and ways to get vitamin D through sunlight and diet

The Endocrine Society recommends all women be screened for vitamin D and that ideal blood levels are **30–50 ng/mL** (75–125 nmol/L). Note the two different methods of measurement—ng/mL is more commonly used.

The best way to get this hormone we call vitamin D is through sunlight, but lack of time, unsafe outdoor environments, indoor work, overuse of sunscreen, certain religious and dietary practices (such as veganism), and pollution make getting healthy sun exposure and D at the right time and in the right amounts difficult. Darker skin, damaged or aging skin, obesity, and pregnancy are all characteristics that increase needs for D, yet these populations are not screened for D deficiencies routinely.

For light-skinned people, daily sunlight exposure on bare skin in 20- to 30-minute increments between 10:00 a.m. and 2:00 p.m. in the middle latitudes of the United States (35°N to 40°N) during the months from April to October will get your vitamin D levels up. Note that during winter months in the north and middle of the US, the sunlight is not at the right angle to give you the exposure you need, so getting exposure in other times of the year is important to get your levels up when the sunlight is available. More sun exposure is needed for darker-skinned women, since greater amounts of melanin in the skin slows or blocks this process of D synthesis in response to sun exposure. A very dark-skinned person might need 40 minutes or more of exposure. The percentage of skin exposed also affects vitamin D synthesis—just hands and face (approximately 10% exposure) would require more time for adequate D synthesis than if more skin was exposed.

Some foods have vitamin D, and you should incorporate them into your diet regularly, especially during the winter months when you can't get the sunshine you need. Those foods include salmon, sardines, tuna, egg yolks, mushrooms, and cod-liver oil. Some foods are frequently fortified with D, such as cow milk, soy milk, and cereals. It is healthier to get vitamin D from foods naturally high in D rather than relying on fortified foods, which are not as healthy and might have added sugars or be a source of digestive difficulties, such as dairy. If you can't afford fresh fish, canned fish is fine and is good on top of salads and/or bread. Try to eat more of those foods during your pregnancy and while breastfeeding.

Foods high in vitamin D

My favorite way to get vitamin D through salmon or sardines is to have them on top of a salad. You can use this recipe for a starter and tailor it to your preferences. I like to use the very affordable prewashed, cut, and bagged curly kale instead of the more expensive salad greens; plus, it is so easy since it is already washed and cut. I just remove the big ribs of the kale for salad. I also love mixing arugula and red cabbage with the kale. Add the salmon or sardines, toasted pumpkin or hemp seeds, grated cheese, and finely cut-up leeks or red onions. Or use homegrown greens and arugula during the growing season! Dress simply with olive oil and balsamic vinegar to taste. This salad is good for many of the other nutrients I discuss in this book. NOTE: These are approximate measurements—tailor measurements to your preferences and availability of ingredients.

• RECIPE: SALAD WITH SARDINES •

- 1 cup of curly kale, precut/prewashed
- 1 cup salad greens of your choice (I use arugula for its tangy taste)
- 1/4 cup finely cut-up red cabbage
- 1/4 cup finely sliced leek or onion
- 1/4 cup cut-up dried or fresh fruit (I use dried mango without preservatives)

- 1/4 cup toasted pumpkin seeds, nuts, or hemp seeds
- 4-ounce can sardines packed in olive oil (which you can use as part of the dressing)
- Olive oil from the sardines, or 1–2 tablespoons extra-virgin olive oil (if you want to decrease fish taste)
- 1–2 tablespoon(s) balsamic vinegar
- Salt, pepper, and seasonings to taste

Cut up the greens into bite-size pieces. Mix all ingredients together and season to taste.

Sardines are a nutrient-dense seafood with protein, many essential vitamins and minerals, and anti-inflammatory omega-3 fatty acids. Sardines eat plankton, so they don't carry heavy metals and toxins like many other fish do, thus they're one of the cleanest seafood sources. Sardines can be bought fresh or in a can and are another easy addition to the pantry for both protein and vitamin D. They are also more affordable than other fish. **Kale**, a member of the cabbage family, is another nutrient-dense food with vitamins (especially K and C), beta-carotene, minerals including calcium and magnesium, antioxidants and flavonoids, and fiber. It is also very affordable. **Arugula**, with its peppery taste, is also a member of the cabbage family and nutrient dense. It is high in vitamins K, A, C, E, folate, potassium, calcium, and fiber. Both kale and arugula would be prohibited if a person is taking the prescription drug warfarin/Coumadin, but hopefully that is not a prescription pregnant women and mothers are on.

— 2 —

Zinc

Zinc is an essential trace mineral/nutrient needed for enzymes to do their work in our body. These vital functions include DNA formation, cellular growth, protein building, healing of damaged tissues, and immune system functioning. Zinc is very important to facilitate immune responses to infections (including COVID-19) by preventing out-of-control inflammation. It is also important for healthy skin integrity and wound healing. A zinc deficiency usually accompanies other nutrient deficiencies and can cause a loss of taste, smell, and appetite.

The recommended dietary allowance (RDA) for adults is 11 mg a day for men and 8 mg for women. Pregnancy and lactation require more: 11 mg and 12 mg, respectively. The Tolerable Upper Intake Level (UL) is the maximum daily intake unlikely to cause harmful effects on health. The UL for zinc is 35 mg daily for adults.

Importance during pregnancy and breastfeeding
Zinc is especially needed to support periods of rapid growth and development, such as during pregnancy/fetal life and

babyhood, because it helps cells to grow, multiply, and differenti-
ate. Adequate zinc levels are necessary for the activity of enzymes,
processes such as mitosis (cell duplication), synthesis of DNA
and protein, and gene expression and activation. These primary
physiological roles of zinc during periods of rapid growth and
development prove its importance during pregnancy and breastfeeding. Pregnant and breastfeeding women and children are
the most vulnerable groups to zinc deficiency, and deficiencies
during pregnancy have ill effects on maternal/fetal growth and
infant birth weight. Zinc also plays a critical role in the oxytocin
binding protein. Studies show that zinc creates a structure that
allows oxytocin to bind, and without zinc, you do not get the full
benefit of oxytocin signaling, which is important in childbirth
and breastfeeding. (More about oxytocin in Chapter 5.)

Symptoms, conditions, and problems related to deficiencies
Conditions and signs of zinc deficiency include skin lesions,
skeletal abnormalities, hair loss, night blindness, anorexia, diarrhea, growth restriction, slow wound healing, depressed immune
function, taste and smell impairment, and neurobehavioral
changes such as lethargy and depression. Fertility problems or
trouble getting pregnant could also be a sign of zinc deficiency. Advanced maternal age, a smoking habit, drinking alcohol,
infections, trauma/stress, and high iron supplementation can
all cause reduced maternal plasma concentrations of zinc and
result in poor transport of zinc to the growing fetus. Fetal life is
a time of rapid growth and development, so a lack of zinc during
pregnancy can be especially concerning. Screening and supplemental zinc is a good idea for women with any of these issues.

Women are generally more often zinc deficient than men, and pregnancy increases the risk of zinc deficiency. Supplementation of folic acid, calcium, and iron (these are in prenatal vitamins) and diets high in cereals/phytates lower the absorption and bioavailability of zinc during pregnancy and can lead to zinc deficiencies. Zinc absorption is notably lower in impoverished communities, likely due to the prevalence of heavily processed or cereal-based diets. Copper-dominated food and water supplies also cause an imbalance of a healthy zinc–copper ratio (15 mg of zinc per 1 mg of copper). Although copper is also important, elevated copper and depressed zinc is one of the most common trace metal imbalances. It is the ratio of copper to zinc, rather than the absolute amount of copper or zinc in the body alone, that makes it possible for enzymes to function properly. Zinc deficiencies also lead to gastrointestinal problems because zinc is an essential trace metal for bacteria of the intestinal flora. In fact, approximately 20% of dietary zinc intake is used by intestinal bacteria.

Depression is more common with zinc deficiency because of altered gut function and the mind-gut connection. Studies have suggested that zinc deficiency increases the risk and severity of depression, and supplementing zinc improves mood as well as cognitive function. Some scientists are even saying that zinc deficiency can be a marker for mood problems. Mental health is so important for motherhood, and the incidence of prenatal and postpartum depression is increasing, so zinc sufficiency should be assessed to avoid these conditions.

Since zinc also supports the immune system, mothers and babies with deficiencies are more at risk for infectious diseases.

Maternal zinc deficiency has also been related to complications during labor and delivery that may affect pregnancy/fetal outcomes, such as prolonged labor, hypertension, postpartum hemorrhaging, spontaneous abortion, and congenital malformation.

Zinc is also needed for every stage of lactation—initiation, continuation and milk production, and involution (weaning). It has been noted that mildly zinc-deficient rats made less milk, so complaints of low milk supply and baby's slow weight gain could be a sign of zinc deficiency and need evaluation. Zinc is also needed in sufficient amounts to fortify a breastfeeding mother's milk for her rapidly growing infant. Sometimes a mother may lack a necessary enzyme that is needed to metabolize her zinc into her milk, but that is rare; mostly, just a general zinc deficiency is the problem. A breastfed infant's growth and development could be stunted if a breastfeeding mother is low in zinc. Zinc is at least as deserving of the attention that is given to folic acid, calcium, and iron during pregnancy.

Current prenatal policy and practice
It has been estimated that as much as 40% to 80% of all pregnant women worldwide suffer from zinc deficiency, but this issue is also not studied thoroughly enough. During pregnancy, it is recommended that women should absorb 3 mg of elemental zinc per day, which translates into an intake of 15 mg of zinc per day. Higher dietary intake or supplementation needs to be considered when lower absorption is an issue due to the situations described above.

There is no routine zinc assessment for pregnant women, since it is assumed that the prenatal vitamin will cover their zinc needs. Most prenatal vitamins have zinc in them; however, many pregnant women are nauseated and unable to take their prenatal vitamins regularly in the first trimester. This means they are lacking enough zinc during this critical early prenatal/fetal period of growth and development. Also, the fact that prenatal vitamins always have iron and calcium in them also means that the zinc in them will not be well absorbed.

Assessment, sources, and supplementation

Clinical (dietary assessment by RD) and lab assessment of maternal zinc status and providing supplemental zinc to correct insufficiencies are prudent to help reduce the high premature birth and infant mortality rates in the USA, decrease childhood diarrhea and respiratory infections, and enhance growth and development among at-risk infants. Clinical assessment can then be used to guide supplemental need. Breastfeeding mothers also need assessment for zinc deficiencies since their milk needs to have a good amount of zinc for their rapidly growing babies.

Prenatal vitamins are very inconsistent and unregulated in both the types and amounts of nutrients they contain, yet most OB doctors prescribe them to all their clients as if they are a panacea for all pregnant women's nutritional needs. When zinc is included in prenatal vitamins (not all prenatal vitamins have zinc in them), it is usually 11–15 mg, a small dosage. Prophylactic doses of 20–25 mg of elemental zinc per day have generally been used in pregnant women in developing countries. The World Health Organization set the upper level of zinc supplementation at 35 mg zinc per day. Care should be taken not to oversupplement with too much zinc (as is true of any supplemental vitamin). Again, the best way to get nutrients is through whole foods, but if there are risks for or signs of a deficiency, then a consultation with a dietitian and/or doctor would be wise.

Foods high in zinc

Like vitamin D, zinc from animal sources is the most easily absorbed form. Oysters are very high in zinc, but few women eat oysters regularly, and women are counseled to not eat raw fish/oysters during pregnancy. Cooked oysters are available canned and are good with multigrain crackers for a snack.

Meat, shellfish, and dairy are foods high in zinc, so vegetarians and vegans might be at risk for lower zinc levels. Nuts and seeds (pumpkin seeds especially) are good sources of zinc. Commercial cereals are often supplemented with zinc, but the phytate levels in cereals and grains complicate zinc absorption. Legumes also have high phytate levels even though they are also a good source of zinc. Oats are high in zinc and fiber.

Adding pumpkin seeds to salads and/or oatmeal is a great idea. Pumpkin seeds are also high in fiber and magnesium. Oats are a good source of zinc, fiber, and nutrients for milk production during breastfeeding. A good recipe for breakfast is oatmeal; it is better to use whole oat "groats," steel-cut, or old-fashioned oats rather than highly processed oats. Adding fruit and pumpkin seeds or nuts and milk of your choice makes a delicious vegetarian and low-cost breakfast rich in fiber, vitamin D, and zinc.

• RECIPE: GROATMEAL •

- 2 cups groats (whole oats with hulls removed)—you can substitute steel-cut oats
- 1/2 cup pumpkin seeds

- 1/4 cup dried figs—the figs will add the sweet taste so no need to add extra sugar
- 1/2 cup fortified milk type of choice

Rinse the groats or oats and just cover with water. The evening before, bring them to a boil and let stand overnight. The groats should be cooked enough and just need heating up in the morning. Toast the pumpkin seeds at 250°F in a toaster oven for 15 minutes and let cool. Cut up and add figs, toasted pumpkin seeds, and your milk of choice to the groats/oats for a delicious and hearty breakfast.

— 3 —

Magnesium

Magnesium is another essential mineral/nutrient that is vital to health and especially important during pregnancy and motherhood. Magnesium through the diet comes mainly from the ingestion of leafy green vegetables, whole grains, nuts, and fish. It is required for regulation of body temperature, nucleic acid and protein synthesis, and nerve and muscle cell function. It has an important role in modulating vasomotor tone, blood pressure control, and cardiac function because it relaxes muscles and dilates vessels. Magnesium is needed in proper amounts to balance vitamin D, vitamin K, and calcium and is also important to mental well-being. A deficiency can result in increased irritability and anxiety. Magnesium is needed in proper amounts to help correct commonplace vitamin D deficiency, as discussed in Chapter 1.

Causes of magnesium deficiency include inadequate dietary intake, eating highly processed foods, poor absorption and/or increased losses through the gastrointestinal tract or kidneys, and increased requirements for magnesium, such as in pregnancy. Older age, diabetes, high alcohol intake, gastrointestinal illnesses, and surgery also increase the needs for magnesium. Taking calcium supplements can cause an imbalance in magnesium, and most prenatal vitamins have calcium in them.

Magnesium deficiency is prevalent in the United States due to foods grown in poor-quality soil, as well as highly processed and chemicalized diets, especially among low-income families. Widespread uses of glyphosate, fluoride, and chlorine in farming cause foods to be low in magnesium. Diets heavy in sugar, caffeine, and high-calcium dairy are also causes of magnesium insufficiency. Digestive disorders and diabetes, which are common ailments in the United States, increase the need for magnesium and the risk of deficiency.

Importance during pregnancy and breastfeeding
Magnesium is needed for a healthy pregnancy and fetal well-being: It supports fetal growth and bone formation, promotes maternal energy, relaxes muscle tension, helps the pregnancy to continue to term, and regulates blood sugar, cholesterol, vascular tone, and heart rhythm.

Magnesium is one of the most important co-nutrients for vitamin D metabolism and is also important for oxytocin hormone function, which is needed for birth and breastfeeding.

The need for magnesium increases during pregnancy, and many pregnant women do not meet this increased need, so pregnant and breastfeeding women are at greater risk for magnesium deficiency. Nausea and vomiting in pregnancy, food aversions, and lack of fresh foods make it hard for pregnant or breastfeeding women to consume enough magnesium through their diet.

Symptoms, conditions, and problems related to deficiencies

Low magnesium during pregnancy has been associated with miscarriage, preterm birth, preeclampsia, and even birth defects. Many less serious but common symptoms during pregnancy could be related to magnesium deficiency, such as fatigue, constipation, swelling/edema, high blood pressure, problems sleeping, and anxiety. Studies have cited links between magnesium inadequacy and conditions in pregnancy associated with mortality and morbidity, such as gestational diabetes, preterm labor, preeclampsia, cerebral palsy, and small for gestational age or intrauterine growth restriction. Magnesium deficiency during pregnancy may pose a health risk for both the mother and the newborn, with increased incidence of lifelong metabolic and cardiac disease and osteoporosis.

Current prenatal policy and practice

Pregnant and/or breastfeeding women need around 350–400 mg per day of magnesium. Research has shown that extra magnesium supplementation has reduced prenatal and birth complications, but there is no consistent policy for assessing or supplementing prenatal/maternal magnesium. Prenatal vitamins have no consistent amount of magnesium or type of magnesium. Some kinds of magnesium supplements are more bioavailable than others, and other types are used to treat constipation and are not well absorbed.

The risk of magnesium deficiency and need for assessment and/or supplementation for childbearing women do not receive enough attention from the OB medical establishment. The incidence of preeclampsia and preterm births are on the rise in the United States and could be related to magnesium deficiencies during pregnancy. The medical treatment for the serious issue of preeclampsia is to administer magnesium sulfate by IV, so it stands to reason that ensuring adequate magnesium in prenatal diet and/or supplementation might help prevent pregnancy-related high blood pressure and preeclampsia. It has been suggested by some researchers that hypomagnesemia may be a marker for true preterm labor.

Assessment, sources, and supplementation

The most widely used method for determining magnesium levels is the serum magnesium test, but it has significant limitations. Clinical dietary assessment by a registered dietitian is most often not utilized until there is already a problem, but it could be, and should be, utilized as part of routine prenatal care. Common prenatal vitamins are very inconsistent in the amount of magnesium they have, with a range of 0–50 mg listed in some popular vitamins, yet 50 mg is only 13% of the RDA.

Magnesium supplementation during pregnancy when a deficiency is suspected or noted by clinical assessment may be able to reduce fetal growth restriction, preeclampsia, and preterm birth and increase birth weight. Magnesium supplementation is generally harmless even if there is not a diagnosed deficiency, and it also can help pregnant women to suffer less from constipation associated with pregnancy and postpartum, as it acts as a laxative in some forms. In fact, constipation is one common symptom of magnesium deficiency, and many pregnant women suffer from constipation at some time in their pregnancy.

There are calls for the further study of magnesium levels in pregnancy and improved screening and testing to avoid prenatal and birth complications. Pregnant women should be clinically assessed for dietary magnesium sufficiency and counseled to increase their intake of magnesium-rich foods such as nuts, seeds, beans, and leafy greens and/or to supplement with magnesium at a safe level.

Foods high in magnesium

Magnesium occurs widely in many foods: greens, whole grains, legumes (especially black beans), vegetables, nuts and seeds, fish, and avocados. It is therefore not surprising that magnesium deficiency is less likely in healthy and well-resourced individuals who eat fresh and varied diets. However, food processing and use of herbicides containing glyphosate (such as Roundup) lead to marked depletion of magnesium in food sources. Low-income pregnant women are at greater risk due to fresh and organic foods being more expensive than processed foods. Unfortunately, many processed foods are subsidized by our government—more so than fresh and organic foods—and therefore, they are unnaturally cheaper.

Some of the vegetables highest in magnesium are spinach, Swiss chard, kale, avocados, lima beans, and squash. Pumpkin seeds (also high in zinc), chia and hemp seeds, almonds, and cashews are all high in magnesium. Many legumes, such as beans, are good sources of magnesium. Salmon is the best high-protein source of magnesium (and vitamin D also); fish is higher in magnesium than chicken or other meats. Dark chocolate is also high in magnesium!

Organic foods are best for magnesium, as glyphosate herbicides used by conventional farmers significantly reduce magnesium levels in foods. Glyphosate is used in several applications during the growing process by all conventional wheat farmers, with the last application being right before harvest, and it has a negative effect on our gut flora as well.

• RECIPE: AVOCADO SALAD AND DRESSING •

Adding avocados to any green salad, as a toast topper, or with a black bean and kale taco is a wonderfully nutritious and easy way to boost magnesium levels. Avocados are a wonderful food and can be used in so many ways. They are usually tolerated well by pregnant women and are a good source of healthy fats and calories.

Just add half an avocado to your favorite salad. Also add black beans or chickpeas, toasted pumpkin seeds, and/or cashews (for added zinc and protein as well as magnesium).

Or use avocado in salad dressing:

Blend 1 large avocado, 1 clove peeled garlic, 1/2 tablespoon fresh lime, 3 tablespoons olive oil, and 1/4 teaspoon salt and pepper (or to taste).

• RECIPE: AVOCADO TOAST OR SANDWICH •

Spread half an avocado on top of toasted, organic, whole wheat or sprouted wheat bread and top with spinach or greens of choice, thinly sliced red onions, and seasonings of choice. Add another piece of toast to make a sandwich if desired.

— 4 —

Fiber

Fiber is a very important nutrient for maternal nutrition and healthy gut flora (intestinal microbiome). Fiber increases intestinal motility and normalizes bowel movements by increasing the weight and size of your stool and attracting water to soften stool. It helps to maintain bowel health by feeding the good bacteria in your gut so you have a healthy microbiome necessary for the assimilation of other nutrients. Fiber also controls blood sugar levels and lowers cholesterol levels. Importantly, fiber aids in achieving healthy weight before and during pregnancy. Fiber helps people chew, digest, and feel full, so it tends to decrease caloric intake. Processed foods have low fiber unless they are supplemented, but natural fiber from foods is much healthier. Water is needed in sufficient amounts to help fiber do its work.

Several types of fiber need to be included in a woman's diet during pregnancy and breastfeeding. **Insoluble fiber**, **soluble fiber**, and **prebiotic fiber** are all essential to our health and well-being.

Soluble fiber aids digestion by attracting water turning to gel. Soluble fiber is found in foods such as nuts, seeds, beans, barley, oat bran, lentils, peas, and some fruits and vegetables, as well as the common fiber supplement psyllium. Soluble fiber helps lower risk of heart disease and diabetes by lowering cholesterol and blood sugar levels. **Insoluble fiber** does not dissolve in water and is found in foods such as the bran of whole grains and beans, the stalks and cores of vegetables, and seeds and nuts. It is not broken down during digestion and is not a source of calories. It adds bulk to the stool and helps food pass more quickly through the gut. **Prebiotic fiber** feeds your gut microbiome. These non-digestible food fibers have a beneficial effect by stimulating the growth of good bacteria in the gut. This creates a healthy gut flora and aids digestion.

Fructooligosaccharides, galactooligosaccharides (natural sugars), and inulin are examples of **prebiotics**. Prebiotics feed the probiotics in the gut. **Probiotics** are the healthy bacteria that populate a healthy gut. They aid in digestion, nutrient absorption, and nutrient production and provide protection from toxins.

Importance during pregnancy and breastfeeding

Pregnancy is a time when healthy fiber is especially needed to offset the common complaints of gastric motility problems: nausea, gas, burping, reflux, and constipation. It is also needed to help regulate blood sugar and insulin levels, decrease gestational diabetes risk, prevent too much weight gain and obesity, and lower blood pressure and cholesterol levels for heart health. Excessive prenatal weight gain and gestational diabetes are both associated with too little fiber, so increasing fiber and fluids can help to moderate prenatal weight gain and manage prenatal blood sugars.

It is important for the mother to have a healthy intestinal/ gut microbiome since her gut flora will have a big influence on her baby's health. Babies need exposure to the maternal gut flora, and they get this through vaginal birth. Fiber, with its natural prebiotics to feed the healthy bacteria, can help correct imbalances in gut flora before birth.

During breastfeeding, low milk supply could be another symptom related to slow intestinal motility, and fiber and fluids will help with this problem. That might be why oatmeal and whole grains are said to increase milk production because they are full of fiber. In fact, most galactagogues (milk production enhancers), which increase milk production for mothers who have a low milk supply, stimulate gut motility as well. We do not fully understand and have not researched the link between gut motility and milk production, but there seems to be an association. It stands to reason that eating more fiber and adequate water consumption would help milk production in breastfeeding mothers. Oats, veggies, other whole grains, and teas with fenugreek and fennel are recommended for increasing milk supply—and they all stimulate gastric motility. The medicines used as galactagogues, such as Reglan or domperidone, are also gut motility stimulants.

Symptoms, conditions, and problems related to deficiencies

It is estimated that around 90% of Americans do not get enough fiber. Most Americans get only around 15 grams of fiber in their daily diet. The recommendation is 25–30 grams per day. The United States' history of overconsumption of dairy and meats in our diet has set the stage for gut dysbiosis and constipation due to low fiber intake. It is now recognized that gut health is integral to general health and well-being, and poor gut health is involved in many diseases, including mental illnesses. Lack of dietary fiber sets the stage for many chronic illnesses from metabolic diseases, including heart disease, obesity, diabetes, and cancer.

Constipation is a common problem in the United States and is indicative of our poor gut health. Diarrhea is another form of gut dysbiosis, and many people alternate between the two problems. Increasing fiber actually helps to solve both problems. The rate of healthy intestinal motility is indicated by having a bowel movement once a day and up to three times a day if the gut is functioning well. The poops should be soft, formed, and easily and quickly passed. The color of poo will reflect what you have been eating, so if you eat a lot of greens, you will see a green tinge—and beets cause red poos! A good way to study your own gut motility is to eat beets for dinner; the red color should be visible in your morning poo if your intestinal motility is good. (Note: You will also see red in your urine after eating beets.)

Current prenatal policy and practice
ACOG recommends 25 grams of fiber daily for pregnancy, but that is the normal recommendation for all adults. There is very little information about fiber's ability to prevent and offset the gastrointestinal discomforts of pregnancy. It would make sense to increase recommendations for fiber during pregnancy, since additional calories are recommended for most pregnant women's diets, as well as additional water to go along with the fiber. The

different types of fiber should be considered and balanced in the diet.

Interestingly, all the galactagogues (foods, herbs, and medicines that stimulate milk production) have features that stimulate gastric motility in addition to increasing the hormone prolactin. So it might be that slow gastric motility or constipation is a risk factor or somehow involved with low milk production. This would be another reason to add fiber and water to the postpartum diet, in addition to relieving the discomforts associated with pregnancy.

Assessment, sources, and supplementation

Start by aiming for around 30 grams of fiber per day (15 grams per 1,000 calories) during pregnancy, or more as tolerated along with the extra calories needed for pregnancy. Early pregnancy, complicated by nausea and vomiting, can make it hard to get the needed nutrients, including fiber, so frequent, small meals help. Late pregnancy makes it hard to get enough fiber when the belly is big and only little amounts can be eaten at a time, so smaller, more frequent meals are also important during later pregnancy. Women need to gradually increase their fiber and water intake to allow for the body to get used to it.

A registered dietitian can assess the amount of fiber in a woman's diet and make recommendations for how to increase fiber. Psyllium husk (which is mostly soluble fiber but also has mucilage, which is insoluble) is the most widely used fiber supplement. It comes loose or in a gel capsule. I think the loose form is best; start with small amounts and drink a full glass of water with it, increasing slowly until you achieve the desired results. Many women do not need as much as is recommended on the package, so experiment with what works for your individual system. That means if you use the capsules, you need to open them up and just use a portion in the beginning. Also, using it in the loose form makes it absorb the water more effectively. Be aware that it is often combined with a flavor that has sugar or artificial sugar, so I think it is better to buy it from a health food store in bulk so you can get it without all those additives. Just start with 1 teaspoon (which is approximately 5 grams of fiber), or even 1/2 teaspoon per day, mixed with a whole glass of water and increase as tolerated to the dosage you think is best for you, *considering how much fiber you are getting from your foods*. It is best to take psyllium when you are not taking other supplements, as it can interfere with absorption, so taking it at bedtime is what most people do, assuming they take their vitamins in the morning. Ground flaxseeds or chia seeds can be used instead of psyllium for added fiber.

Healthy ways to eat fiber

Fiber—all types—is high in all vegetables, fruits, legumes, nuts, seeds, and whole grains; it is low in animal-derived foods, such as meat and dairy. So the best way to get enough fiber is to just eat more unprocessed veggies, fruits, beans, nuts, seeds, and whole grains. It is important to drink enough water with fiber-rich foods to help fiber do its work and increase intestinal motility. If you have not been eating that much fiber, it is best to increase fiber intake gradually to avoid symptoms of gas and bloating. Dandelion greens are high in fiber, with 3.5 grams per 100-gram serving, including inulin, a prebiotic fiber. Garlic, onions, leeks, oats, flaxseed, apples, bananas, and asparagus are all high in healthy fibers, including prebiotics.

A diet with adequate fiber should include four to seven servings of minimally processed veggies and two to three servings of fruit per day—more during pregnancy. Fibrous veggies and fruits with skins and membranes are rich in fiber. Beans, lentils, or peas should be eaten three times per week. Snack on nuts, seeds, or roasted chickpeas, or add them to salads, oatmeal, or yogurt. Avocados have a lot of fiber and magnesium and can be used in so many ways: as guacamole dip, a toast topper, or added to sandwiches, salads, or tacos. Choose whole grains like brown rice, wheat flour, and whole groats instead of white rice, white flour, or quick oatmeal. Remember to drink plenty of water to aid the fiber in its work—around 3–4 ounces per hour is a guide, or around 10–12 cups of water for pregnant or breastfeeding mothers.

Eating FRESH for FRESH health is important, especially during pregnancy and breastfeeding. Eating foods naturally high in fiber decreases many symptoms of digestive and gut problems, such as bad breath, dental decay, oral/tongue soreness, nail abnormalities, skin rashes, weak bones, achy joints, headaches, constipation/diarrhea, dysbiosis (bad gut flora and gas/bloating), reflux, and fatigue. Making these healthy nutritional changes during your pregnancy is also important for the health and energy needed for parenting!

Foods high in fiber

Any of the previous recipe ideas will also work for increasing fiber. Note that avocados (a fruit) are high in both fiber and magnesium, and fresh fruits (especially raspberries) and vegetables are both high in fiber and other nutrients discussed in this book. So making fresh foods the biggest portion of your meal will increase your fiber intake as well as the other important nutrients.

• RECIPE: BUTTERNUT SQUASH CHILI •

- 1 medium butternut squash
- 1 tablespoon olive oil
- 2 onions, 1 red bell pepper and 3 cloves of garlic
- 2 cans black beans
- 2 cans diced tomatoes
- 1/4 cup chili powder
- 1 teaspoon cumin
- 1 teaspoon cinnamon
- 1 tablespoon unsweetened cocoa powder or 2 squares of 75% dark chocolate
- Sugar and salt to taste
- 2 cups brown rice

Toppings as desired:
- Scallions
- Cilantro
- Red onion or leeks
- Grated cheese
- Diced hot peppers
- Greek yogurt

Peel, seed, and cube butternut squash (or buy prepped/frozen). Toss butternut squash in a bowl with 1 tablespoon olive oil and 1/4 teaspoon salt and bake at 400°F for 30 minutes. Slice onions, bell pepper, and garlic, then sauté them. Separately, drain and rinse black beans.

Mix baked squash, onions, bell pepper, garlic, black beans, tomatoes (undrained), chili powder, cumin, cinnamon, cocoa powder/dark chocolate, and sugar and salt in a large pot and simmer for at least 30 minutes.

Cook brown rice.

Serve chili with cooked brown rice and top with finely chopped scallions, cilantro, red onion or leeks, grated cheese, or diced hot peppers. You can also add a dollop of Greek yogurt as desired.

— 5 —

Oxytocin

Massage to increase oxytocin is another nourishing factor/nutrient for pregnant and breastfeeding mothers, and for partners and babies too. It is important for general health and well-being and even more important during pregnancy, childbirth, breastfeeding, and parenting. Massage helps both *the recipients and the givers* relax, decrease stress, relieve and distract from pain, enhance circulation, and, importantly, enhance **oxytocin**, the hormone needed for birth, breastfeeding, and bonding. Massage stimulates both oxytocin production and receptor function. Oxytocin is both needed in and enhanced by loving relationships and communication, sex, childbirth, breastfeeding, bonding, and human touch. Women giving massage to their partners and babies also helps, so *giving massages* (when there is energy to do so—not during childbirth or immediate postpartum!), not just receiving them, is beneficial.

Oxytocin is often called the "love" hormone because it is released when one engages in any sort of physical, social, loving, or sexual contact. The release of oxytocin during sexual activity allows the couple to enjoy a stronger bond, which is important to

45

relationship health. Oxytocin is produced by the hypothalamus gland and secreted by the pituitary gland (master gland). I also like to refer to oxytocin as the "movement hormone" because it helps things flow in the body by producing contractions—in the uterus, intestine, breast, and other vessels. It is a pulsating hormone, so the rhythm of uterine contractions and the flows or "letdowns" of breastfeeding are due to rhythmic oxytocin pulses.

Importance during pregnancy and parenthood

Oxytocin plays an important role in the human body and behaviors of both sexes, especially in women during pregnancy and lactation. Oxytocin levels increase during pregnancy and especially during labor, with increasing size and frequency of pulses of oxytocin. Large pulses of oxytocin occur during birth and breastfeeding, stimulating uterine contractions, breast ductal contractions, and even intestinal contractions (that's why women have to poop often in early labor).

Oxytocin moves the milk from mother's breast to baby and is very important in the mother's milk production, even though it is not the hormone that makes the milk (which is prolactin). The milk will not be made if the breast is too full, so oxytocin is needed for the milk to leave the breast and enable prolactin to do its job to make the milk.

More oxytocin is released when there is a trigger such as skin-to-skin embrace, touch or massage, or baby's suckling or crying, and even a loving smile or communication can cause higher releases. When the mother starts breastfeeding, oxytocin is released, allowing milk to be released from the breast. Oxytocin is produced and secreted in response to every breastfeeding.

Oxytocin released within the mother's brain influences maternal physiology and behavior during birth and breastfeeding. It helps inspire loving parental behavior and helps parents cope with the demands of parenthood. The release of oxytocin very importantly deepens the bond between mother and child and helps the mother to act lovingly toward her needy (and sometimes annoying) infant. Women who go through natural labor (versus a planned C-section without labor) and who breastfeed have higher oxytocin levels, so they get more of this behavioral benefit.

Oxytocin also has effects on intrauterine brain development and future behavior of a child. Studies have shown that people with higher oxytocin levels are more socially connected and tend to communicate better even when there is a problem. It is an important hormone for physical as well as neurological, behavioral, and mental health. It has been noted that people with autism have lower oxytocin levels.

Using massage to stimulate and enhance this very important hormone, oxytocin, is an effective and pleasurable method of self-care. Also, getting a professional massage is wonderful for mothers but can be expensive. Gift certificates for massages are a good idea for gifts for new parents! The nutrients I have discussed previously in this book also help oxytocin production and function during pregnancy, childbirth, and breastfeeding.

Symptoms, conditions, and problems related to deficiencies

Oxytocin levels are usually only measured in research studies and not in the usual prenatal care setting. Therefore, low oxytocin levels are mainly identified by symptoms. Deficiency symptoms include little to no pleasure during sexual intercourse, stress, social detachment, anxiety, depression, aggression, stalled labor during childbirth, and breastfeeding problems, including low milk production and problems with milk flow.

Nutrient deficiencies of magnesium, vitamin D, and zinc can be a reason for inadequate oxytocin production and function, as I stated before. Fiber has not been studied as it relates to oxytocin, but it is known that stimulation of intestinal motility, as fiber does, is somehow connected to enhancing lactation (galactagogue effect). So it might be assumed (and definitely deserves study) that a low-fiber diet and constipation are somehow connected with low oxytocin levels.

Stress and pain interfere with oxytocin. Lack of skin-to-skin contact with a baby who is hospitalized or otherwise separated from the mother results in poor oxytocin production and function. Single motherhood and lack of a loving, intimate partner can be involved in poor oxytocin function. Not breastfeeding or weaning early from breastfeeding causes oxytocin production to decrease.

Current prenatal policy and practice

Unfortunately, most OB practices and policies do not attend to the need for touch, massage, or movement during labor and delivery to enhance the expression of natural oxytocin. Instead, Pitocin (an artificial oxytocin hormone) is used to compensate in most OB labor and delivery settings. Currently, Pitocin is used around 30% of the time to induce (start a labor) and is also used to augment labor when it slows down after a woman has an epidural. Almost 70% of women receive epidurals, which slow labor and then lead to higher Pitocin usage. Pitocin is also given after most deliveries to prevent uterine hemorrhage postpartum. So there is a lot of Pitocin usage.

Birthing centers with doulas (professional labor support people) and midwife-attended home births facilitate oxytocin expression by using massage and other ways to naturally support laboring women. It would be better if OB care incorporated more massage during childbirth to increase natural oxytocin production; then maybe the use of artificial Pitocin could be decreased.

Assessment of problems resulting from high Pitocin usage

Artificial oxytocin (Pitocin) given during and after childbirth as an infusion does not cross into the mother's brain because of the blood-brain barrier and does not influence brain function in the same way as oxytocin during normal labor. Artificial Pitocin also acts to fill the oxytocin receptors and blocks natural oxytocin's function for a while after the Pitocin is given. So a woman who received a lot of Pitocin during labor might have a delay in her own oxytocin and milk production.

Sources of oxytocin: Massage and breastfeeding

Daily massage during pregnancy, childbirth, and breastfeeding is a pie-in-the-sky sort of recipe but a worthy goal. It would be so nice if insurance covered getting professional massages during pregnancy, childbirth, and breastfeeding! Doulas, trained and certified in labor support, are also trained in massage techniques for childbirth, pregnancy, and postpartum. Doulas can work with you and your partner, giving and also teaching you massage methods to use at home. It would be wonderful if all OB services also staffed doulas as part of the labor and delivery services. Some (but few) insurance companies cover doula costs. Doulas are well worth the expense, as they reduce complications and interventions during childbirth, thereby reducing medical care costs. I used to work at a hospital where a grant funded doulas for women in childbirth who wanted them.

Partners can give each other massages using gentle and loving touch methods like hugging, kissing, stroking, rubbing, rocking, tapping, pressing, cupping, etc.—all techniques you can incorporate in massage or loving touch during lovemaking, pregnancy, childbirth, and breastfeeding. Even making good eye contact increases oxytocin expression and feelings of trust.

The massages do not have to be long; try getting or giving them in small increments—a back rub in the morning, maybe a longer massage before bedtime, hugs and kisses here and there. Massage for the baby helps to calm and comfort them when they are fussy, and it is a gentle form of sensory stimulation that aids neurological development. Massaging the baby's belly gently also helps when they have gas or colic symptoms.

Getting a massage of the shoulders before or during a breastfeed helps moms to release their milk (have letdowns) so the baby gets the milk sooner and easier. This is especially helpful in the early days of breastfeeding, when moms have tension, nipple soreness, and other postpartum discomforts. Pain stymies oxytocin release, and massage can counteract this.

Gentle breast massage and compression also helps to move the milk from the breast and prevent or treat milk stasis or clogged ducts. Hand expression of milk involves the use of massage to bring the milk down toward the nipples so it can then be expressed. Adding gentle breast massage/compression to breastfeeding helps the premature/less-efficient baby get more milk per feed and save their energy, and it also aids a mother's milk production. All mothers need to learn how to do breast massage and expression.

Massage, breastfeeding, nipple stimulation, and skin-to-skin contact are all natural and effective ways to increase your oxytocin levels. Oxytocin is so important for many health reasons, but especially for birth, bonding, and breastfeeding! The nutrients I have discussed in previous chapters and massage all work to enhance the oxytocin function.

Summary of Nutrients and Foods

I have chosen potent nutrients and foods to highlight in this book. These nutrients are important for healthy pregnancy, breastfeeding, and parenting. Massage as an oxytocin enhancer is included as a "nutrient" important for pregnancy, breastfeeding, and parenting.

Here is a summary of the foods and their nutrients/effects:

- **Pumpkin seeds**—zinc, magnesium, fiber, protein, healthy fats, B vitamins, and iron; good for immunity, growth, energy, and healthy blood sugar
- **Nuts**—protein, fiber, low glycemic index; slows sugar absorption when eaten with other foods
- **Sardines or salmon**—protein, omega-3 fatty acids, vitamin D; good for pregnancy and fetal growth, bone development, and immunity
- **Oats/groats**—zinc and fiber; good for lowering blood sugar and and maintaining a healthy weight
- **Butternut squash**—fiber and magnesium, carotenoids (a nutrient that is associated with yellow, orange, or red vegetables or fruits and is an antioxidant that protects

cells from damage of toxins), and vitamins B and C; low calorie but dense in nutrients and usable in so many ways

- **Kale/spinach/dark leafy greens**—fiber, calcium, magnesium, and vitamins C, K, and A; good for pregnancy, gut health, blood sugar, and immunity
  - **Curly kale** is the most common type. The bright green leaves look like ruffles.
  - **Dinosaur kale** has narrow green leaves that are wrinkly like dinosaur skin. The leaves are attached to a firm stem that should be removed.
- **Avocado**—healthy fats, fiber, and magnesium; good for energy and growth
- **Onion/leeks/garlic**—inulin (prebiotic fiber); good for gut health and flavoring
- **Dried fruit without extra sugar added (prunes/apricots/figs)**—fiber, magnesium, and other vitamins. Dried fruit is high in sugar and should be used sparingly to naturally sweeten meals or for a snack combined with nuts, which slow the absorption of their sugar. I've chosen these dried fruits because they are lower in sugar than some of the other dried fruits.

Finally, massage is so important and enjoyable! Try to work it into your schedule frequently for its most rewarding and beneficial aspects. Both receiving and giving massages bring you benefits, so do both for health and to strengthen the bonds between family members!

Nurture

In this book, I have focused on what mothers can do to nourish and nurture themselves and their babies. I hope you have gotten some good ideas on how to nourish yourself to sustain breastfeeding more easily. I have written another book, *The Recipe for Breastfeeding Support in America*, in which I discuss the breastfeeding support mothers deserve but do not receive. In that book, I focus on how our country, health care system, and policies need to improve breastfeeding support to increase mothers' success with breastfeeding. Mothers are being given the message "you should breastfeed" but are not given the support they need to do that easily. I make recommendations for system changes and also for what mothers themselves can do to gain more breastfeeding support.

The following poems and photos with mothers' messages are meant to inspire you to choose and sustain breastfeeding, which is the healthiest way to *nourish* and *nurture* your baby. It is also very empowering for you, the mother, and improves your health.

Breastfeeding is hard at times but so worth the effort. It is good work that has lasting impact. It is sometimes hard to keep on breastfeeding when you are experiencing difficulties and pain or losing your milk production. My hope is that reading these poems and knowing other mothers have struggled and sustained breastfeeding will help you to be strong and carry on with breastfeeding! Partial breastfeeding is very good too, so even if you aren't able to fully breastfeed, it is worth it to keep on partially breastfeeding. It is the best gift you can give to yourself and to your babies. You will always be proud of your work breastfeeding.

Messages From Breastfeeding Mothers

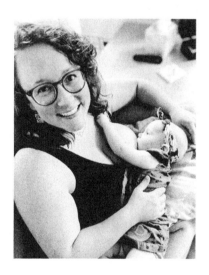

"Breastfeeding my children has been one of the most rewarding and empowering experiences of my life. It's been a lesson in patience, communication, perseverance, and surrender—these are powerful life teachings, and I'm so grateful to have had the opportunity to learn from my body and my children in this way."

—*Ashley Tysh (she/her), La Leche League member*

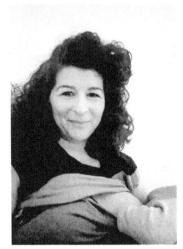 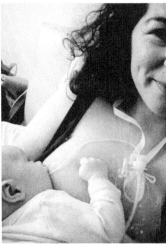

"Even an untypical breastfeeding journey can be a success-
ful one! Having supply issues, with the help of a supplemental
nursing system, I was able to breastfeed my son past 10 months.
Despite all the challenges we had, he still loves the breast and
finds comfort in it."

—*Cristina Kerr, La Leche League member*

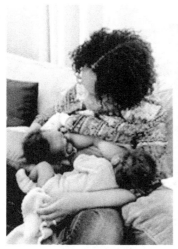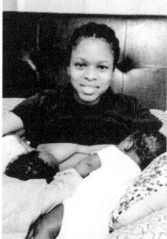

"Every day that I feed these little ones, my ideas about what is possible and feasible are stretched. They grow and grow, and as they do, I'm able to surround them with so much love, provision, and comfort. I think about the women before me who fed generations from their bodies, and I join them with so much gratitude!"

—*Stephanie Godwin-Chu, La Leche League Leader*

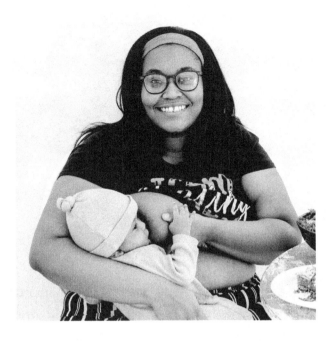

"Breastfeeding to me means health and connection. I'm so thankful for the ability to lactate."

—*Xanielle Rodgers and DeAndre Iman*

Breastfeeding Poems

It's Mom's Secret Recipe
by Erin L. O'Reilly, 2015

It's Mom's Secret Recipe
Oh, So Fine
Specially Formulated
Every Time

It's a Feat of Biology
Nature's Art
A Womanly Superpower
From the Heart

This Potent Elixir
Of Liquid Might
Nourishes and Protects
It's So Right

This Corporeal Effusion
Of Good Health
Endows Our Children
With a Wealth of Health

Nourish with Your Milk
And by Your Breast
It's as Strong as Silk
Endures All Test

This Wholesome Brew
From Mother to Child
Through Ages and Cultures
Tames Our Wild

Hundreds of Ingredients
Known to Be
For Each Babe It's Customized
All for Free

Even Through Turmoil
Trouble or Strife
Breast Is the Very Best
For a Good Life

This Gift Everlasting
Is a Liquid Glue
Bridging and Bonding
Me to You ♡

The Gift

by Erin L. O'Reilly, 2021

This Gift of Luscious Liquid Love
From Mother to Child
Most Pure, and So Rich
From a Strong Mother with Soft Breast
Sweet and Salubrious
Tastefully Nutritious
Solid in Benefit, yet Gently Given
This Warm Fluid Love
A Helping of Hardiness
In a Unique Recipe of Universal Love
Flowing to the Future
From the Here and Now ♡

Sustaining through Sustenance

by Erin L. O'Reilly, 2020

Breastfeeding... a Sustaining Sustenance
Even in an Era of Dearth and Death
Connection, Communication, Communion
Sustained during Disability and Disconnect
Heterogeneity to Counter Extreme Homogeny
Consumption of Flora-Filled Fluid
From Mother's Breast to Baby's Body
Bacterial Biome Lining Baby's Belly
Versus Sterility Imposed by COVID
Immunity Passed, and Inspired
Stem Cells from Mom's Milk to Baby's Brain
Protecting, Growing, Developing
Enriching, Enhancing, Enticing
Tasteful Even in a Tasteless Time
A Nurturing and Fine-Tuned Therapy
A Way of Sharing during Separation
Socializing Baby while Social Distancing
Opportunity for Smiling amid Masking Mandates
Satisfying in Time of Great Dissatisfaction
Rich Even during Economic Deprivations
Empowering while Restrictions Disempower
A Womanly Art amidst Pandemic Science
Healthy in Spite of a Tsunami of Infirmity
... Breastfeeding ♡

The Milky Way of Breastfeeding

by Erin L. O'Reilly, 2019

They are as on a magical journey
Mom and breastfeeding Baby
Winding through the Milky Way

The come and go
The up and down
The flow and dribble
The more and less
The fore and hind

Always changing and full of variety
Each time a new recipe
The intimate exchange of flora and fauna

The letting-go and taking-on
The past and present
The here and now
The history and future
The ancient and modern

This Nourishing and Nurturing
Lacteal fluid we call milk
Mammalian treasure trove of protection

From Mother to Baby
For Baby to grow and develop
For Child to immunize
For Society to protect
For Humankind to continue ♡

Liquid Love

by Erin L. O'Reilly, 2021
A poem of Ls in honor of La Leche League's enduring legacy of mother-to-mother, worldwide breastfeeding support for the past 65 years.

Lacteal Lady-Lager
Liquid Love
DeLicious and deLightfuL
Logical and Longevous
Lofty Liquor
Mother Lode of Love

LollapaLooza Mamma
Luminary Mother
Laboring to yieLd
LiteraLLy succuLent
LegitimateLy saLubrious
PowermiLk of heaLth

Little one Longing and Lingering
In Momma's LapLand
Lusting for Luscious,
Leaking, even Leaping
Lacteal Lubricant
So deLicousLy deLivered

Lick-abLe and LikabLe
Lunch of Love-age
Linchpin and Lucky charm
Lipid-fiLLed Lactation
Living and Lasting
Lush mammaLian Liturgy

LimitLessLy fLuent and affLuent
FLowing fLuid
Luscious and iLLustrious
Luxurious Liniment
Lacteal Liquid
Like white bLood

LiveLihood of a Live-bearer
Legendary Leche
LocaListic and Laureate
LaicaL and LiabLe
LiberaLizing Lager of
Lactiferous Motherhood

LadyLike yet Lion-breasted
La Leche League Leaders
Long Legacy of heLp
Latching Babe to Mom
Linking past to present
Leading to a Luminous Later ♡

About the Author

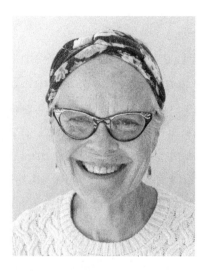

I LOVE my work spreading light and love through the empowering, health-promoting work of breastfeeding support!

Thank you for taking an interest and reading my book *Nourish and Nurture: Overlooked Ingredients and Empowering Poetry for Pregnancy, Breastfeeding, and Motherhood!*

—Erin L. O'Reilly, RN, MSNR, IBCLC

Erin L. O'Reilly is an RN, master of science in nursing research (MSNR), International Board Certified Lactation Consultant (IBCLC), volunteer La Leche League Leader, retired WIC breast-feeding coordinator, public health nurse, past president of the St. Louis Breastfeeding Coalition, and member of the Missouri Breastfeeding Coalition, the US Breastfeeding Coalition, the United States Lactation Consultant Association (USLCA), and the International Lactation Consultant Association (ILCA, ilca. org). She lives and works with the breastfeeding community in St. Louis, Missouri.

During her time as president of the St. Louis Breastfeed-ing Coalition, she helped to get a Missouri state breastfeeding law passed, obtain 501(c)(3) status for the coalition, and plan and fund the Breastfeeding Photo Project in 2014; helped write a grant for funding to start the I AM: Breastfeeding support group led by leaders in a Black community in St. Louis; and participated in many World Breastfeeding Week events over the years and other community events. She has been a volunteer La Leche League Leader since 1999 and has led over 3,000 meetings as a Leader, taken countless phone calls, gone on many home visits to moms needing help with breastfeeding, and trained and certified many new La Leche League Leaders to continue the work of breastfeeding support. Erin taught childbirth and breastfeeding classes and worked in the lactation department of a major hospital in St. Louis for 19 years; she worked in the Nutrition and WIC Department in a neighborhood health care center as a breastfeeding coordinator from 2007 to 2020.

Erin's breastfeeding support experience has encompassed a wide variety of situations, and she has worked with many different women who have many different breastfeeding experiences, barriers, and/or supports. She breastfed her own son as well and personally experienced the barriers to breastfeeding, which inspired her to become a La Leche League Leader and an IBCLC to help others have an easier time on their breastfeeding journeys.

Contact Erin at **ErinLOReilly.com**.

Looking for more information about breastfeeding and pregnancy? **ErinLOReilly.com** has valuable resources and beautiful artwork, plus a link to buy Erin's book *The Recipe for Breastfeeding Support in America*.

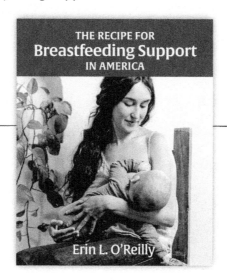

Made in the USA
Monee, IL
24 July 2023

39854964R00046